# The SMART SNACK

## *The No-Hunger Way to Lose Weight*

### David Bell

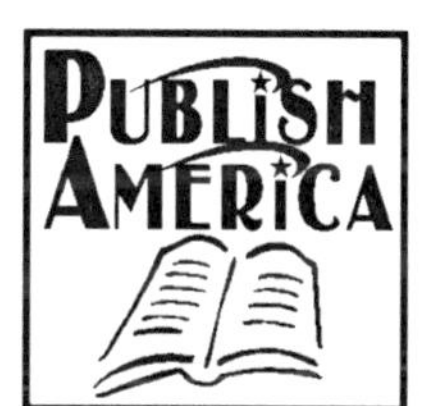

PublishAmerica
Baltimore

ISBN: 978-1-60749-703-5 (softcover)
ISBN: 978-1-4489-2258-1 (hardcover)
PUBLISHED BY PUBLISHAMERICA, LLLP
www.publishamerica.com
Baltimore

Printed in the United States of America

# Introduction

This book *is* one man's experience with successful weight loss. Your author does not have an M.D. degree but does have a doctor's degree in a related medical field. The book is the result of personal experience and much research of medical literature and medical treatment. This book does not read like medical literature, however; it is simplistic by design, so that anyone, especially school children, would be able to read and understand it.

# Chapter I

It is obvious that we are overeating and putting on too much weight. For a long time I've thought we were eating too much "fast food" and consuming too many calories. It is true that a double burger with large fries and a large soft drink will probably zoom past one thousand calories. But, also, the food industry has tempted us with many delicious cookies, crackers, chips, and combinations that are hard to resist. The food industry has reduced the fat content of many of the cookie and cracker creations, but the public seems to be gaining more and more weight. Primitive peoples do not have weight problems because they have to perform more physical work and do not eat refined foods.

# Chapter II

There have been recent discoveries in medical research that shed some light on the causes of obesity and hunger. Of the three food types—proteins, carbohydrates, and fats—fats have been taking the blame for the problem. However, fats as well as proteins, have a complicated route of utilization; they go from stomach to intestine to blood stream to the liver where it changes them *into* thousands of enzymes and other chemicals. Carbohydrates are much more simply utilized. Carbohydrates are changed to glucose (blood sugar) in the stomach and intestine and are our source of fuel in the blood stream. This blood sugar can be utilized immediately, or stored as glycogen for future use or stored as **FAT**. The hormone insulin is necessary for the blood sugar to enter muscle cells and to be stored as fat. So when more carbohydrate is consumed than is necessary for exercise. it is stored as FAT.

# Chapter III

If eating too much carbohydrate foods leads to more fat in our bodies, then we need diets that have fewer carbohydrates (carbs for short). One of the first low-carb diets was devised 150 years ago by a Paris physician who was treating his diabetic patients and found that they lost weight on his diet plan. A London physician soon adopted the same diet and also had success in helping patients to lose weight.

In 1972 Dr. Atkins proposed his low carb diet; in fact, it was almost a no carb diet. He sold millions of books over the years, but few people could or would continue with his diet. There was much criticism from the medical profession of Dr. Atkins saying that it was all right to eat as much fat as one wanted.

The South Beach Diet by Dr. Arthur Agatston came on the scene in 2003 to wide acclaim and great acceptance. This diet is similar to Dr. Atkins in that it is a low carb one, but it does not suggest unlimited consumption of fat. The South Beach program does start with absolutely no carbohydrates for the first two weeks.

Both of these diets have been difficult for people to continue because of the body's hunger mechanism. When one's blood sugar gets too low, the brain sends hunger signals. Hunger may be somewhat satisfied by eating bulk, protein, and fat (because they may be slowly converted to blood sugar), but feelings of hunger are best satisfied by small amounts of carbohydrates.

# Chapter IV

Until 1994, the American Diabetes Association and physicians treating diabetes recommended that diets should severely limit all sweets and that so-called complex carbohydrates (starches) would be fine to eat in large amounts. But medical research has shown that starches are actually very quickly converted to glucose or blood sugar and have the same dangerous consequences as sugary foods. So, in 1994, the American Diabetes Association recommended the restriction of all carbs as well as foods containing large amounts of sugar. The diet schools that teach diabetic patients how to measure the carbs they eat are doing a better job than any diet plan to date. But they still haven't come up with a satisfactory suggestion for snacks. That important topic will be addressed in Chapter VII.

# Chapter V

Most of us are probably not aware of the variety and number of carbohydrate foods that we eat every day. We need to list all the carbohydrate groups in order to measure and limit our carb intake:

1. Bread and grains. Also includes breakfast cereals, pancakes, waffles, rice.

2. The potato family could be included with vegetables, but we separate the many varieties for emphasis. We must be on the watch for the many casseroles, baked, new potatoes, and, of course, French fries.

3. Snacks are also separated. Com chips and popcorn could be included with grains; crackers and cookies could be as well. Of course, potato chips are a major snack.

4. The vegetable group is interesting in that many vegetables are so low in carbohydrate count that they are considered free; there is no need to measure carbs in a green salad. Peas, beans, and com must be measured, though.

5. Fruits are an important carbohydrate source. Unlike the vegetable family, all fruits must be measured and counted.

6. Sweets, of course, must be counted. Some desserts pack a gigantic number of carbs. Yet some chocolate candies don't have as much carbohydrates as might be expected. Carbs *must* be counted.

7. The dairy family includes milk, milk shakes, ice cream, sour cream, yogurt, and cottage cheese, but does not include cheese.

8. Beverages to be included are regular colas and soft drinks but not diet colas. Light beer does have less than half the carb content that regular beer has.

9. Combination foods, such as macaroni and cheese, are difficult to estimate. Soups, stews, chili are in this group, and their content labels must be read. This type of restaurant food is always a carbohydrate mystery, and must be consumed in limited amounts.

# Chapter VI

Now let's look at meal planning from a low carb standpoint. Breakfast and lunch will be easier than dinner because the customary menus are more limited.

Most people will choose from a breakfast menu offering of cereal, toast, eggs, bacon, sausage, pancakes, fruit, or waffles. You wouldn't or couldn't eat some of each category, so count your carbs and limit yourself to a small bowl of cereal with milk, a small bowl of fruit, and some eggs and lean bacon. If you should choose cereal, milk, fruit, toast, you would exceed your carb limit of two carbs for women or three carbs for men (one carb is equal to 15 grams). A bowl of cereal with milk is two or three carbs; so any additional selections should be from non-carb groups such as eggs and bacon or sausage. Toast, two pieces, will be at least two carbs, so no cereal or fruit should be eaten, but eggs and bacon would be fine. Bagels seem to be high in carbs, so one should limit a portion to half a bagel and add eggs and bacon. The same can be said for pancakes and waffles. The point of being selective is not to be hungry but to limit the carbohydrates and eat more protein to be satisfied.

When lunch time comes, the choices are again clear cut. The bread in a sandwich is the main if not the only source of carbohydrates in a sandwich, be it lettuce and tomato, ham and cheese, or hamburger. When you choose a side, pick a green salad, rather than French fries. For a beverage, choose a diet drink or unsweetened tea rather than a regular cola. A large salad with grilled chicken or salmon or beef tips would be an excellent low carb lunch.

The dinner choices are more complicated. Soups and casseroles are unknowns; they may have considerable carbohydrates so one must only eat a minimum amount, such as one fourth of a cup, to avoid overeating carbs. Cooked vegetable dishes are also unknowns, especially peas and beans, but they can be usually safely eaten in amounts up to one-half cup. Breads must be compared visually to knowns such as a slice of bread. Of course desserts must be rationed and estimated according to a known such as a candy bar. Cheese cake desserts seem to be the carb content champions; just be warned. You know by now that meats, fish and salads are considered to be carb-free.

# Chapter VII

We have finally arrived at the most important weight-loss section—the snack. Let's face it—low carb diets probably leave everyone hungry after two or three hours. Knowing how to snack will make the difference between success and failure.

Remember it was previously mentioned that the hormone insulin utilized the blood sugar after a meal into energy for muscle movement, glycogen for energy storage, and also into fat if there is blood sugar left over. When the body detects new glucose entering the blood to become blood sugar, it sends signals for a surge of insulin to utilize the glucose and reduce the blood sugar level to a normal range of between "80 and 120." When blood sugar level is down near the 80 area, hunger signals are sent out.

Recent research revealed that a snack or meal of four grams or less of carbohydrates would not trigger a surge of insulin flowing into the blood stream. The four grams is enough to relieve the hunger sensations but not enough to cause a new flood of insulin. That means a snack of four grams or less is truly a SMART SNACK! The four gram snack can consist of several olives (up to twenty); or a few nuts (must be measured, of course); or some sunflower seeds. You may count out four Pringles potato chips (one gram per chip) or any favorite cracker or cookie, as long as it only measures four grams or less. Sometimes I eat a regular green salad which will usually have less than four grams of carbohydrate. My very favorite smart snack is one peanut butter cracker (NOT an entire four or six cracker packet)—just one cracker.

This snack may be eaten about two to three hours after a meal of 30 grams of carbohydrate. If a person is exercising or doing yard work or active housecleaning, you may need a second or third smart snack in thirty to forty-five minutes. The need will vary according to the exercise. This is why marathon runners will pick up a paper cup of juice or Gatorade during a race.

# Chapter VIII

Exercise is, of course, very important in weight control. The conventional wisdom is that one should exercise for one hour three times each week. Shorter workouts are discouraged because the heart rate may not be elevated enough. We will present a different view because of the effect exercise has on blood sugar levels. Remember that insulin utilizes blood sugar as fuel in muscle movements and storing glycogen and fat. Exercise acts as an insulin substitute by removing blood sugar that would otherwise be stored as fat. Diabetic people are told that it is preferable to exercise for twenty to thirty minutes between meals so that their blood sugar can be kept in a low, normal range most of the time. This method will total to more exercise time and help even more to control weight. Sixty to ninety minutes each day is to be preferred over three hours of exercise per week. *Walking* is the most important exercise. Moderate arm and weight exercises should also be included. Walking can be done almost anywhere; inside one's house works just as well as outside walking.

# Chapter IX

To sum everything up, let's remember that low carbohydrate diets are not new, that they date back at least one hundred fifty years.

Dr. William Harvey of London wondered if obesity and diabetes might have the same cause. His patient, Mr. Banting, was five feet five inches tall and weighed 202 pounds. Dr. Harvey put him on a diet: no potatoes, bread, butter, milk, sugar, or beer. Mr. Banting lost 46 pounds in less than a year. His menu was meat or fish for breakfast. At lunch he ate fish, vegetables and fruit. At dinner he dined on the same plus two glasses of red wine.

# Chapter X

Even back then it was recognized that overeating carbohydrates is what leads to weight gain. There are so many carbohydrates to choose from in the grocery store that it is difficult not to over eat them. Think how many aisles of a store are dedicated to high carb food: soft drinks, crackers and cookies, potato chips and pop corn, canned fruit, breads, dairy, deli, sweets, and ice cream, as well as combination foods. All these foods can be eaten, but must be measured to prevent over eating them.

Over eating carbs also makes us hungry. The surge of glucose (blood sugar) entering the blood stream causes a surge of insulin into the blood stream to utilize the blood sugar by causing it to be stored in the muscles as glycogen or as fat. So we need to be doubly careful about over eating carbohydrates.

Close examination of the menus at our many fast food restaurants reveals the probable reason for American obesity. Most items are heavy laden with carbohydrates. If someone wants to lose weight at a restaurant, there are only a few choices—a salad of some kind. All the sandwiches, fries, large drinks, and desserts are carbohydrate heavy. In the last thirty years the fast food restaurant business has multiplied eighteen times.

A low carbohydrate diet is essential for control of diabetes and will result in weight loss as well, if it is adhered to. To just vaguely aim at a low carb meal is not sufficient; the carbohydrates consumed must be measured and must not exceed thirty grams per meal for women and forty-five grams per meal for men.

The snack is even more important for success in weight loss. The smart snack must not exceed four grams at one time; it may be repeated in forty to sixty minutes, depending on the amount of exercise during the time period.

The recommended exercise is simple walking with the addition of moderate arm and weight exercises. Rather than longer, less frequent exercise periods, it is recommended that one walk twenty to thirty minutes between meals and after the evening meal.

Low carbohydrate diets are well-known for being difficult to stay with for any length of time. Using *smart snacks* will make the adjustment easier. It may also be helpful for the first two weeks for women to eat forty-five grams of carbohydrates per meal; after two weeks the carbohydrate amount should be lowered to thirty grams per meal. For men the carbohydrate amount may be sixty grams per meal for the first two weeks before lowering the amount to forty-five grams per meal.

Some more discussion is needed about combination foods and dairy foods. Many of these foods are misleading in appearance concerning their carbohydrate content. When a food contains two major types of carbohydrate, such as cake or cheese cake, the total carb content may be surprisingly high. Ice cream and some other dairy products are in this category too. You will need to read a lot of these nutrition fact labels until you are familiar with them.

The benefits of losing weight can't be praised enough. You will feel better in general. You will have more energy. You will feel better about the way you look. That should be enough, but you will definitely improve many aspects of your health.

Good luck and best wishes!

# Chapter XI

Here is an easy to remember way to get started and it may be all that you need.

1. Limit sweet eating to *two* bites.
2. Eat no crackers, potato chips, cookies, popcorn, corn chips, except in four gram amounts.
3. No soft drinks with sugar or chocolate milk.
4. No potatoes, French fires.
5. Eat only one sandwich.
6. Salads are unlimited with smaller portions of meat or fish.

If loss of weight does not seem to be happening along with the suggested amount of exercise, then more exacting carbohydrate counting needs to be started.

In any situation a snack should only be a smart snack size.

# Credits

The South Beach Diet         Arthur Agatston, M.D.

Wall Street Journal         Cynthia Crassen, 5-5-04

Keeping Well With Diabetes

     Pennington, Jean A. Bowes and Church's Food Values of Portions

     The Food Processor ® Nutrition Analysis and Fitness Software

American Diabetes Association      www.diabetes.org

The Complete Book of Food Counts   Corinne T. Netizer

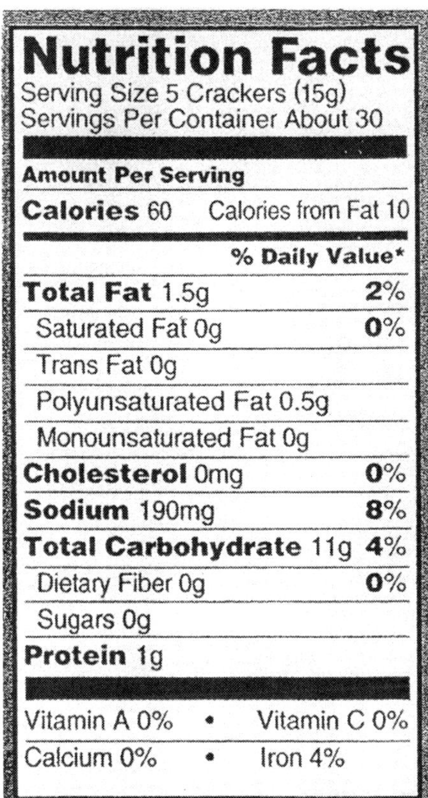


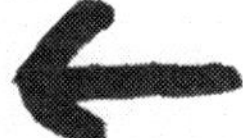

How to read nutrition labels:

The only listing we really need to read is the total carbohydrate amount (arrow). This label from a saltine cracker box shows that five crackers have eleven grams. So for a smart snack, only two crackers may be eaten. Crackers eaten with a meal (maybe with soup) must be counted so that total carbs for the meal won't exceed thirty to forty-five grams.

# Carbohydrate Content of Foods

| Food | Size of 15 gram portion (1 carb) |
|---|---|
| **(1) Breads & grains** | |
| Whole wheat loaf | 1 slice |
| White loaf | 1 slice |
| Cereals | |
| Oat cereal (cheerios) | 1 cup |
| Raisin Bran | ½ cup |
| Crackers | |
| Saltines | 8 crackers |
| Rolls—dinner | 1 roll |
| Bun—hamburger | one equals 1 ½ carbs |
| Hotdog | one equals 1 ½ carbs |
| Waffles | one equals 2 carbs |
| Rice-brown | 1/3 cup equals 1 carb |
| Instant | ½ cup equals 1 carb |
| Pancakes | 1 4-inch |
| Muffin | ½ muffin |
| Biscuit | ½ biscuit |

(2) Vegetables

| | |
|---|---|
| Beans—green | 2 cups |
| Lima | ½ cup |
| Red kidney | ½ cup |
| Beets | 1 cup |
| Broccoli | 2 cups |
| Carrots—raw | 2 cups |
| Cooked | 1 cup |
| Celery—cooked | 2 cups |
| Raw | free |
| Corn-on-cob | 1 ear |
| Canned | ½ cup |
| Lettuce | Free |
| Mushrooms | 2 cups |
| Okra | 2 cups |
| Peas-fresh | 1 cup |
| Canned | 1 cup |
| Frozen | 1 cup |
| Radishes | free |
| Spinach | 2 cups |
| Squash—summer | 2 cups |
| Tomatoes—raw | 2 cups |
| Canned | 2 cups |
| Tomato juice | 1 cup |
| Tomato sauce | 1 cup |
| Turnips | 2 cups |
| Turnip greens | 2 cups |

(3) Fruits

| | |
|---|---|
| Apple | 1 apple |
| Applejuice | ½ cup |
| Applesauce—no sugar | ½ cup |
| Apricots | 3 |
| Banana | ½ banana |
| Blackberries | 1 cup |
| Blueberries | 2/3 cup |
| Cantaloupe | 1 cup |
| Cherries | 20 cherries |
| Dates | 2 dates |
| Grapefruit | ½ grapefruit |
| Grapefruit juice | ½ cup |
| Grapes | 15 grapes |
| Orange | 1 orange |
| Orange juice | ½ cup |
| Peach | 1 peach |
| Pineapple | 1 cup |
| Plum | 1 plum |
| Prunes | 3 prunes |
| Raisins | 2 tbsp |
| Raspberries | 1 cup |
| Strawberries | 1½ cups |
| Tangerines | 1½ tangerines |
| Watermelon | 1 cup |

(4) Dairy

| | |
|---|---|
| Cottage cheese | ½ cup |
| Sour cream | 1½ cup |
| Ice cream | ½ cup |
| Milk-whole | 1-1/3 cup |
| Non-fat | 1-1/3 cup |
| 1% | 1-1/3 cup |
| Yogurt—low fat | 1 cup |
| Buttermilk | 1-1/3 cup |
| Chocolate milk | ½ cup |

(5) Beverages

| | |
|---|---|
| Beer | 12oz (1 carb) |
| Light beer | has ½ carbs |
| Carbonated drinks: | |
| Diet soda | free—no carbs |
| Cola | ½ cup |
| Fruit flavored soda | ½ cup |
| Ginger ale | ½ cup |
| Root beer | 1/3 cup |

(6) Combination Foods

| | |
|---|---|
| Beef stew | 1 cup |
| Chili con came | ½ cup |
| Macaroni & cheese | 1/3 cup |
| Pizza | 1 slice |
| Spaghetti with meat sauce | 1/3 cup |
| Soups | |

| Beef with vegetables | 1½ cups |
| Chicken noodle | 1½ cups |
| Clam chowder | 1 cup |
| Consommé, beef | 3 cups |
| Consommé, chicken | free |
| Cream of chicken | 1½ cups |
| Cream of mushroom | 1½ cups |
| Split pea | ½ cup |
| Tomato | 1 cup |

(7) Potatoes

| Baked | 1/3 potato |
| French fries | 10 fries |
| Mashed | ½ cup |
| Scalloped | ½ cup |

(8) Crackers, cookies

| Crackers (saltine | 8 crackers |
| Cookies (2 inch) | 1 cookie |
| Fig bar | 1 bar |
| Potato chips | 15 small chips |
| Popcorn (popped) | 3 cups |
| Candy bar (1 oz) | 1 bar |

(9) Sweets

| Cake | 1 Tbsp |
| Brownie | one |
| Chocolate chip cookie | one |

| | |
|---|---|
| Cupcake frosted | ½ |
| Custard | 1/3 cup |
| Honey | 1 Tbsp |
| Jam, jelly | 1 Tbsp |
| Pie | 1 Tbsp |
| Pudding | 1 Tbsp |

# Smart Snacks

(Four Grams)
Amounts

| | |
|---|---|
| Carrots | 4 baby carrots |
| Celery | 1 stalk |
| Frito Scoops | 3 |
| Cheese Nips | 5 |
| Vanilla Wafer | 1 |
| Saltine | 2 crackers |
| Pringle chips | 4 |
| York mint | ½ of one |
| Almonds | 20 |
| Town House Crackers | 2 crackers |
| Triscuit | 1 |
| Wheat Thins | 3 |

# Author Favorites

Amounts

| | |
|---|---|
| Green tossed salad | any size with Wishbone spritzer |
| Pecans | up to ½ cup |
| Olives | up to 20 |
| Peanut butter cracker | 1 cracker |
| Sunflower seeds | 1/3 cup |
| Chiquita Apple Bites | 4 slices |

9 781607 497035